I0416048

Table of Contents

Copyright

From flab to fit without diet or exercise

Written by Sara Marks

Copyright 2012 by Sara Marks

Smashwords edition

About the Author

I've been an expert in the weight loss business for more than twenty years and know what works and what fails with weight loss. Many experts are quick to give medication and diet supplements, but I know there is more to losing weight.

Unfortunately, there are no miracle drugs or any supplements that will magically take off the weight, but there are secrets to making you healthy and lighter than you are now. With this book, you will be successful with weight loss. You will never need another book about losing weight ever again.

Over the twenty years that I've been a weight loss expert, I have learned the guaranteed ways that have helped many lose the weight and keep it off. This book will guide you to weight loss easier than you ever thought it was possible. I have the secrets to weigh loss and I am now sharing them with you.

Join the many that have loss the weight using my secrets. Once you have the secrets, you too will soon be on your way to losing weight and keeping it off for good.

From Flab to Fit without Diet or Exercise

By

Sara Marks

Congratulations! You made the right decision to gain control over your weight.

Trust me. You will not be disappointed with this book. Everything you need to be successful with weight loss is in this book.

Now, I want you to answer honestly to these questions:

✓   Do you often feel tired, bloated, and not yourself?

✓   Do you wonder why you don't have enough energy through the day?

✓   Do you want to know why you just don't feel like yourself anymore?

✓   Are you ready to start losing weight today?

If you answered yes to any of these questions, then this book is right for you. It sounds like your body is not working properly and you need to find a way to regain control of how you are feeling. It might be time to give your body a makeover and a well deserved tune-up with the secrets I have for you in this book.

When your body is carrying the excess weight, you are not working to your fullest potential and you feel tired, lazy, and unmotivated. These problems could be the reason you are always feeling emotional, sad, and uncomfortable every time you walk out your door.

By carrying the excess weight, you are holding yourself back from feeling normal again. There are a number of factors that prevent you from losing weight, but I will guide you through with book to success with your weight loss. You don't have to feel tired, unmotivated, or unhealthy any more.

All you need is an easy-to-understand guide that will make you successful with weight loss and helping you regain your health. Most diet and exercise programs expect unreasonable goals that ordinary individuals cannot reach. Most of us do not have the time or money to spend on diets and exercise programs that just don't work.

What this book will do for you

This is why I wrote this book, helping many succeed with weight loss. This book will give you everything that you need to lose weight without a diet or exercise program. This book will give you everything that you need to be successful with weight loss. You will start to feel better and start to feel more energetic than ever before.

In this book, you will:

✓ Learn the secrets to losing weight the healthy way

✓ How to maintain success with your weight loss

✓ Have control over your weight

✓ Understand how to shed the excess weight without a weight loss program

✓ Understand how weight loss works with the secrets in this book

✓ You will fix the problems that were holding you from feeling like you again

Many have learned the secrets to losing weight and you will too. Join the many who already learned the secrets to losing weight success and start today. After all, what do you have to lose…….except the extra weight.

What you will learn

What I am offering you is the secrets that will make weight loss easier and permanent. The secrets I will offer to you will help you lose the weight and keep it off without an expensive diet or a diet that is difficult to understand. This is not a diet, but changes to how you eat. By changing how you eat, you will soon be on your way to losing weight easily and effortlessly.

What this book contains:

✓ Everything you need to know for losing weight

✓ Easy-to-understand guide for losing weight quicker than any program

✓ Easy-to-follow instructions to losing weight the healthy way

✓ 5 secrets to weight loss revealed

This book will help you easily understand how to lose weight and keep it off. Many who try to lose weight fail because the diet or exercise programs are difficult to understand or have unreasonable expectations for losing weight.

This book contains all the information and secrets to weight loss in one book that is easy to understand and follow, even if you do not have any extra time or money to spend on a program.

What you will not find in this book:

✓ A magical way to lose the weight overnight or in an unhealthy way

✓ Difficult guide that only experts can follow

✓ Promises that cannot be reached

This book gives you easy-to-follow instructions that will help you jumpstart your weight loss and keep you losing weight until you reach your goal. You will never need to use a diet program or medication that will make you feel sick ever again.

Losing weight and keeping it off

All you will need is my top five secrets to losing weight easily, effortlessly, and permanently. The secrets are easy to follow and do not require buying any products or following a meal plan that does not sound appealing.

What I am offering to you is a new way of looking at weight loss, by giving you the top five secrets to making it a reality right now. There are millions of individuals that are overweight and struggle with weight loss, only to gain the weight right back.

This phenomenon is called the yo-yo effect which makes you feel tired, bloated, and uneasy because you are not yourself. Every time your weight fluctuates, your body's ability to work properly is affected. This will cause you to feel unmotivated and unenergetic.

I will give you the secrets to reversing this effect without any effort, giving you the body you want. Learn the secrets to losing weight and you will join the millions who already know each one that I have revealed.

Join the many whom were once looking for the answers to weight loss and now have everything they need to make it true.

What affects weight loss

The ability to lose weight is influenced by several factors in your life. Some factors cannot be avoided, but can be reversed by the choices you make.

I will help you understand what factors affect your success with weight loss in the past. I will also help you understand what you can do to help change your weight loss problems now.

With this book:

✓ You will learn what affects your ability to lose weight

✓ You will understand what you need to fix for weight loss to occur

✓ You will understand how to lose weight

✓ You will learn how to fix the problems with the secrets to weight loss

Losing weight doesn't have to be difficult or out of reach for you. It is possible and you will soon be on your way to losing weight with the 5 secrets to losing weight. First, let's explain the reasons why you are struggling to lose weight.

Understanding the factors that affect your weight loss is important to losing weight. Understanding how to lose weight effectively starts with the problems that are preventing you from losing weight right now.

Reasons why you can't lose weight

Losing weight seems unreachable to many, but I am here to tell you that it is possible. There are many factors that affect the ability to lose weight quickly, but the secrets revealed in this book will allow you to succeed with weight loss. Before I reveal the secrets to weight loss, let's begin with why you can't lose weight right now.

Knowing what affects your weight will help you understand why you are unable to lose the weight. Knowledge is important to winning the battle with your weight. Understanding the reasons for your weight struggles will help you understand how to overcome the obstacles. The more you know, the easier it will be to losing weight.

AGING

> After thirty, your body's metabolism decreases by 5 percent and continues to decrease with every decade that passes. Unfortunately, this is part of the aging process that cannot be stopped.

> With aging, your body's muscle development decreases, affecting your metabolism's ability to maintain optimal performance to help you lose weight.

> The problem with weight loss is that many individuals do not understand this and continue to eat and act as if their body is the same as it was when they were younger.

> Unfortunately, we cannot go back in time, but we can improve the body's ability to lose weight.

GENETICS

> You are your parent's children is true. Some people were blessed with a genetically fast metabolism, while other people struggle to lose weight their entire life.

➢ Your parents play an important part in your ability to lose weight. This is an unavoidable reality because you cannot change genetics.

➢ Inherited traits from your parents make you prone to diseases, give you the body type that you have, and the problems you will unfortunately have to face in the future.

➢ However, genetics does not have to play a part in losing weight. Fortunately, the genetically caused slower metabolism can be assisted with a few minor adjustments to your body.

➢ This book will help you lose weight just as fast as you would with a fast metabolism.

DIET

➢ The types of food and the calories you consume affect the way your metabolism functions.

➢ The choices you make when you choose a meal will determine how much you can lose or how much you gain, create different reactions to your metabolism, and could prevent the foods you choose from converting into energy.

➢ Knowing how to choose the foods you eat and making it simple to follow will help you lose weight easier than the diet plans and programs that you tried in the past.

➢ Choosing the right foods and the amounts to eat will help you lose the weight.

METABOLISM

➢ Your metabolism defines the way that your body uses the energy from the foods you eat. No one wants a slow metabolism or wants to gain extra weight if it can be controlled.

➤ Knowing the factors that affect the way you process food will help you understand what you need to do to control your weight and your slow metabolism.

➤ Check with your doctor to make sure our metabolism is not affect by any underlying medical ailments that require special attention or treatment.

➤ Knowing what affects your health is very important for you to be successful with weight loss.

So what is the good news?

Fortunately, all of these factors can be controlled with the secrets to losing weight that I have for you. Your body can easily become a fat burning furnace without any dieting or exercising. I have been in the weight loss business for twenty years and have learned the secrets to weight loss. I am now giving them to you.

You will soon be on your way to losing weight and feeling even better than you ever did. You will join the many who already know the secrets and are already on their way to their desired weight.

Once you learn the secrets to weight loss, you will be able to:

     ✓   Lose weight without diet or exercise

     ✓   You will feel better than you have before you discovered the secrets

     ✓   You will have a healthy weight program for the rest of your life.

Secret #1: Knowledge

The phrase knowledge is power is absolutely true when it comes to weight loss.

Knowledge is the most important tool that you need to be successful at weight loss. When you know where to begin, where you are with your weight in terms of health, and what you need to lose to reach your goal, you will know where to begin your weight loss.

Many individuals who fail to lose weight often overlook this important step. This is one of the main reasons why weight loss becomes so difficult. If you don't know what you weight and skip the weight assessment, then how will you know what to do if there is no start to your weight loss?

Assessing your health is the first step to losing weight. Finding out where you are starting will allow you to lose weight faster than you imagined. Here are the two items that you need to know before we move to the next secret and start losing some serious weight.

Here's what you need to know before you begin:

> **Your actual weight**

Be honest about this number. In order to make weight loss happen, you must be honest with where to will start. Many individuals lie about their weight, but this number is only for you to know where you will begin. Don't worry……I will not ask.

> **Food journal of everything you eat.**

Again, be honest with the amount of food and what foods you eat every day. This, again, is for you to know how much you are actually eating and what types of food you choose. This is important for you to see what is causing the weight gain. Sometimes, just knowing what you are consuming will help you realize why you are having trouble with weight loss.

Let's start losing weight!

With the information you learn, just remember to continue to document your food intake throughout and weigh yourself weekly. This will help you stay on track throughout the, ensuring you success and awareness of what you are eating.

Unlike dieting, the food journal is intended for you to understand what foods you are consuming and the amounts you eat, making you aware of the choices that may be causing you to gain weight. Again, many individuals do not realize what they eat in a day, causing them to continue making poor choices with food and overeating.

Knowing what you eat and what you can skip as a choice, will help you begin making better choices for meals. It will also help you start eating better than before, making you realize what you are consuming every day.

Secret #2: Cleanse

The next secret that is often overlooked is your internal health. Many individuals who put any effort towards weight loss forget the importance of their internal health that could be preventing them from losing weight.

If your body is full of toxins, then your body will not work efficiently. It is estimated that most individuals are carrying anywhere from 5 to 25 pounds of toxic waste in their colon. This factor plays a negative effect on weight loss, preventing your body from flushing out the excess weight.

Over the years, you probably have eaten pounds and pounds of fried foods, processed foods, and foods that were chemically infested with pesticides. The junk food you ate is most likely still sitting in your colon, causing fatigue, restlessness, bloating, and constipation. Removing any excess toxins will help you start losing weight quickly once your body is working properly.

There are many products that claim they are effective, but I am telling you that they are a waste of your money. You can do an internal cleanse at home, without spending a fortune for products that do not work. Most colon cleansers involve the use of herbs and supplements that are not regulated or approved by the Federal drug administration.

You don't want to harm or affect your health for weight loss. The goal of weight loss is to improve your health, not harm it with any herbs or supplements that can cause more damage. A colon cleanse should be a natural process that does not add any additional complications.

TIP: Simple internal cleanse that you could do at home:

- 1 cup Aloe Vera juice daily for a week

- 8- 10 glasses of water every day

Aloe Vera is a gentle and natural method that is often used for an internal cleanse. While using this product, you may experience a "healing process" that includes bloating, swelling, and fatigue temporarily, but will soon pass as the toxins leave your body. Aloe Vera is available at most grocery stores in the country.

Once the toxins are removed, you will feel better than you did before, returning your body to normal. This will help you begin to lose weight quickly and effortlessly. This is an important part of losing weight. Once the toxins are removed, your body is able to release the rest of the excess that exists, your weight, easier than before.

Secret #3: Choices

Have you ever heard the phrase, "You are what you eat?" Well, this is very true.

Many individuals often forget that what they eat could define what you will become. If the foods you eat are controlling what you can do, then why wouldn't you choose foods that will help you lose the excess weight?

There are many foods that you can choose to help you lose weight, without feeling as if you are on a diet. After all, this is not a diet program. This is your health.

There are choices you can make that support weight loss, without making you feel deprived of the foods you love. There are many foods that you can eat that will keep you satisfied, without making you feel as if you are on a diet.

Three types of foods you need in your diet

Every individual needs three types of food categories in their daily diets that will help them lose weight and keep it off. Here is the list of the types of foods with examples of each that will help you lose the weight quickly and permanently:

Fiber-enriched foods good for losing weight:

- All vegetables (all types)

- All fruits (all types)

- Beans (all types)

Foods that are rich in fiber will help support weight loss and keep your digestive system healthy enough to continue to remove any excess toxins. Foods with fiber will keep your body working properly and help you slim down, all at the same time.

It is recommended that individuals consume 25- 30 grams of fiber in a day to help them manage their weight. Yet, many individuals only consume a third of this every day, making weight loss difficult to achieve.

What many fail to realize is the importance of fiber for helping to release toxins in your body and help you manage your weight. Fiber is important for weight loss to happen. Fiber also controls your hunger and keeps you feeling full longer than any other food after a meal.

Protein-enriched foods good for losing weight:

- Lean proteins chicken, fish, lean burgers, turkey, pork,

- Veggie burgers

- Eggs and dairy

- Nuts and seeds

Foods that are rich in protein will help support lean muscle and help you burn fat quicker as you increase the lean muscle in your body. Protein is required for weight loss, giving you the needed support for your immunity, insulin levels, and support for increasing your weight loss.

It is recommended that individuals consume anywhere from 10 to 30 percent of our calorie intake per day. Yet, many individuals only consume a portion of this, not giving ample support for their body to produce the lean muscle needed for weight loss to occur.

The type of protein you choose will greatly influence your weight loss and weight goals. Quality proteins refer to lean proteins that do not involve any added fats or oils that could affect your weight loss. Any fried foods should be kept to a minimum or removed from your daily intake if you want to optimize your weight loss potential.

Carbohydrate-enriched foods good for losing weight:

- Baked potatoes and baked fries

- Yams and sweet potatoes

- Whole wheat pasta and breads

- Oatmeal

Foods that are rich with carbohydrates give you the energy needed to make it through the day, keeping you moving. This will help you with burning calories throughout the day. Carbohydrates help to balance your insulin levels by slowly releasing energy throughout the day, helping you stay full longer.

Carbohydrates speed up your metabolism and turn your body into a fat burning furnace for weight loss to occur. It is recommended that one-third of your diet includes good carbohydrates that support your weight loss, but many individuals choose the wrong carbohydrates to consume.

Choosing the right foods

One of the important choices that you make while losing weight is the food you eat. Choosing food that support weight loss will help you lose weight quicker. Choosing healthy over junk food will make your efforts to lose weight possible.

If you choose the smarter choices, I guarantee that you will be able to keep losing weight and continue to lose weight until you reach your weight goals. The food choices you make will affect every effort you give to losing the excess weight. It's all about the choices you make that will affect the outcome you receive with the secrets revealed for weight loss to happen.

Secret #4: Control

One of the secrets to weight loss is portion control. This one is often overlooked or not understood by many while losing weight. Portion control is important during weight loss, but it is more important with counting calories, which is not what this book is all about.

Many individuals put aside weight loss because they do not have the time or the tools available for measuring what they eat. Many overlook the importance of portion control when they are eating, causing them to eat more than they should, causing them to gain more weight than expected.

This secret makes portion control easier for you to follow, and making you lose more weight than you could ever imagine. Here is how you can easily practice portion control while losing weight without any tools for measuring the amount of food consumed:

When making any meal, I want you to follow this guide for every meal that you eat. Here goes:

TIP: When creating a meal, follow this guide:

- Fill ½ of a large plate with fruits or vegetables of your choice

- Fill ¼ of a large plate with proteins of your choice

- Fill ¼ of a large plate with carbohydrates of your choice

If you keep this as a guide for all of your meals (breakfast, lunch, and dinner), you will soon be practicing portion control, calorie intake control, and you will start to see weight loss occurring quicker than you did before.

You don't need a fancy calorie counter or any other tool if you follow this guide for every meal that you eat. This will help you control your weight easily, without having to measure or figure out what to eat. This guide will help you shed the weight with this guide.

Secret #5: Review

This secret is very important to losing weight. Many overlook this simple, yet effective process when losing weight. Only 10 percent of individuals who reach their weight loss goal manage to keep it off in the long run. This is because 90 percent of individuals think that they could repeat the patterns that got them overweight in the first place.

When an individual reaches their weight loss goal, they slowly begin to add the bad habits back into their lifestyle, causing them to begin to regain the weight that was loss. The secret to keeping and controlling the weight off is to review your weight loss every week that passes.

This means that you should weigh yourself weekly, continue taking a food journal for your review, and making sure the bad habits do not start taking over. It is easy to fix a few slip-ups and a few pounds, but trying to lose several pounds will put you back to the beginning.

Tip: What you need during your weight loss:

- Journal of the foods you are consuming daily

- Keep tracking of your weight loss weekly

Reviewing every week will help keep your weight under control and allow you to continue to lose weight even after you reach your weight goal. Do not let your hard work go to waste because you forgot the secrets that I revealed. Be part of the 10 percent that maintains their weight well after your goal.

Many individuals that are trying to lose weight fail to look past the weight loss period and to the future. Measuring your weight and keeping a journal of what you eat, will help you understand what you are eating and what is affecting you with controlling your weight.

Conclusion

Weight loss is about changing the habits, the lifestyle, and making a commitment to better health for the future.

It is not about dieting or exercise, but changing the way you look at weight loss.

Maintaining your weight goals well into your golden years and enjoying a healthier lifestyle for the present is what this book is all about. It is your choice to succeed with weight loss and maintaining your health. It is your choice to have that success, now that you have the secrets to weight loss revealed.

Making the choice to learn the secrets was the very first step to making the choice to reach your ideal weight. Now, it is your choice to make the next step and use the secrets that are now revealed to you for weight loss success.

Join the many who already know and succeed with your weight loss. I wish you the best of luck on your journey to finding a healthier and happier you.

www.ingramcontent.com/pod-product-compliance
Lightning Source LLC
Chambersburg PA
CBHW070940290526
45795CB00003B/1086